Preparation For Healthy Parenting

Preparing for the Ultimate Adventure: A Parenting Handbook for First-Time Parents. Practical Tips for a Healthy and Happy Family.

Anita Singh

About Author

Mrs. Anita Singh, Author of **Preparation For Healthy Parenting.**

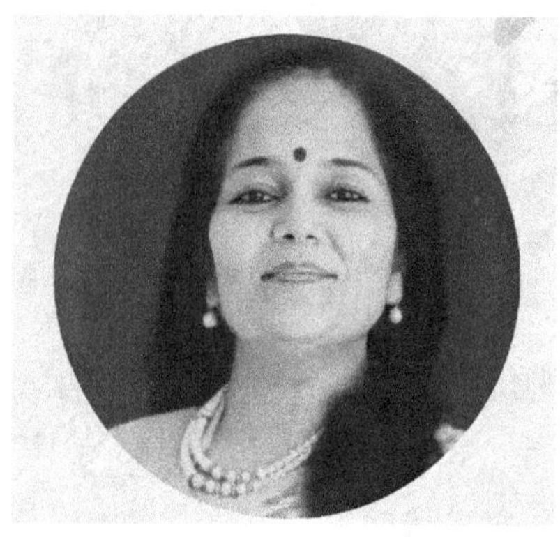

Author of the First Book of the series **'Tips for Healthy Parenting'** of the series of 3 books on the way.

Mrs. Anita Singh was born in **Jammu, India.**

Growing up as an Army Officer's daughter was fascinated with the new places, schools and cultural diversity across India.

Her journey has been exciting and interactions with different people has developed a keen observation into **Behavioural aspects of Parents** towards their **children.**

Anita Singh is a **Trained Postgraduate** English language teacher and has worked in reputed **Army and Public Schools.**

Her experience by working with students and their parents throughout her teaching experience has developed an interest to turn into a **Parenting Coach.**

She is married and blessed with two Angels **Sumedha**(a Clinical Psychologist) and **Abhijeet**(student)

Acknowledgement

Thank you to the **Universe and My Parents** who provided me the education and values to become a prolific writer, **Som Bathla** my mentor has given flight to my wings to fly as an author. I am most grateful to **my family** and especially **my children,** who sincerely wished for and encouraged me to write. Finally, I would mention that I would not have been able to get my work done without continuous support and vision of my editor **Sooraj Achar(#1_BestSeller)** who copyedited this book with enormous skill, warmth and precision.

Dedication

To **My Husband and Children**, for always loving and supporting me and above that bearing with my eccentricity

Contents

Introduction

SHRI Ganpati Namah

"There is no great leadership challenge than parenting." - Jim Rohn

Just like an awesome leader, a good parent will make a child see what he can be, rather than what he is. And the truth is that the best parents desire to serve their children, not themselves. Not practised much in words as in attitude and in actions. To describe parenting a little better, the parents who try to improve their own actions, so that the child inculcates the best. If LOGICAL THINKING is developed at home itself, he will never go wrong. As it is a proven fact that children from well-mannered and sensible families are better citizens of this earth.

Indian Scriptures promulgate a simple rule for parents-

1. From birth to 5 years of age- Treat a child as an Emperor

2. 6 years to 12 years- Inculcate Discipline

3. 13 and above- Treat them like best friends

There is no doubt that parenting is challenging, but remember it is only a phase of life. If these above mentioned years are taken care of, in this way, - Parenting would never go wrong or would never result as a problematic one.

"It Takes a village To Raise a Child". This phrase clicked my attention and I got a Eureka moment to write a book, which opened a plethora of my childhood experiences.

"It took me years to understand, a golden nugget of life- that right behaviour, correct attitude and an amicable approach is all that is required for bringing up a child, and leave the rest for your child to explore".

It is not that, I did not know it but it was only knowledge, but, after getting into the role of a mother, then could I understand that knowledge is not enough to rear a child. It needs a complete personality and a disciplined mindset of a parent, to bring up a child to his/her optimal level.

It Takes A Village: and other lessons children Teach Us is a book published in 1996 by first Lady of the United States- Hillary Rodham Clinton. In it she advocates a society which meets all of the child's needs.

What caught my attention, was this African proverb-

"I takes a village to raise a child."

In my opinion, It is an appropriate one when it comes to raising a child. What I think and have experienced, that an entire community is responsible for providing a safe and healthy environment is needed to develop and flourish.

Each and every experience in the child's life is the sum total of what is happening all around him. The parents, grandparents, siblings, neighbours, teachers, trainers, coaches and religious leaders and others who interact with them during childhood, will have an effect on who your child will be in the future.

There are so many cases in our society itself, where the parents with high values, have gone wrong while rearing their children. We do not always know what our children are learning today and by whom. Before, we could talk about a village as referring to the society but now it is the home environment, people in the school like teachers ,friends etc. and now the internet boom is playing a major role in the lives of the children and parents.

As per the new Positive or Modern Parenting, neither the teachers nor the parents are advocating the 'discipline'. The reasons are considered as following

1. <u>Discipline-too harsh:</u>

-The parents believe that the word 'discipline' is too strict and doesn't fit into an ideal relationship.

The parents also get into a guilt loop-

*They do not want their children to face lots of stress at a young age.

*You were hard on your child a day before.

2. <u>Change in Attitudes:</u>

Parents have changed their attitudes due to many reasons- :

Do not approve of the parenting style of their own parents, or did not approve of their strictness. So, they switched to liberal attitudes to deal with their own children.

3. <u>Fear of Rejection:</u>

In order to avoid conflicts and tantrums, parents are afraid of their kids' reactions. The discipline may result in loss of love with their children(mindset).

4. <u>Lethargic Approach</u>:

To some extent, it is pure laziness on the part of the parents OR they are too tired to deal with their kids, because of their busy schedules.

To take time and deal with the situations related to the child- it needs a lot of enthusiasm and some presence of mind. For them, parenting becomes a burden instead of responsibility or

Those Parents who are not able to stick to the rules, even with the best intentions- the children will take advantage of indiscipline in one or the other form.

5. <u>Low Self-Esteem:</u>

In some cases, it is also observed that the parents with low self-esteem, avoid disciplining the child, at appropriate moments. They themselves go into self- doubt and as a result may take extreme actions to raise their children. As a result, their children sometimes can grow into distorted personalities or may repeat the same patterns as those of their parents.

These people are the ones who raise children, without effort on their part. Today, the world constitutes the majority of such a population which takes life for granted. They stay unaware of the results and take parenting for a ride.

WATCH WHEN YOU ARE SAYING NO
Are you mindlessly saying No to each and everything your child is doing. Instead of telling them what not to do try to convey what to do.

Chapter 1

Preparation to Become a Balanced Parent

"Pay the price, by becoming the person you want to become. It's not nearly as difficult as living unsuc-cessfully. Make your 30 day test, then repeat it, then repeat it again. Each time it will become more a part of you until you wonder if you could have lived any other way. Live this new way and the floodgates of abundance will pour over you."

"You have nothing to lose but you have a life to win"
- Dr. David Harold -MD(West Coast Psychiatrist)

These lines are taken from **'The Strangest Secret of the World'**. I listen to it on a daily basis. I feel blessed to have Siddharth Raj

Shekhar as my mentor who has opened doors of awareness, so that I could come out of my own shell of mental constraints.

What made me go deeper into the sense it conveyed, that if one has the right intentions and strong will, he can even make anything work. I observe these lines to link it to human nature.

"What are we giving our children? Is it money or property? I have seen people work so hard for the money, to give it to the children and then children fight as enemies, to see who gets it. Is that the legacy? Is that a fulfilling life? Is that what we want to leave to the world?

Our values, our character, the grace and the compassion of the love that flows in all of us is the real legacy which as parents we can leave for our children".

Yes, you have got it right. This is what, in a sense, parenting is all about. Some of them would feel tensed, to even dream of having a child and try to start planning well beforehand about their parenthood. The same sense of doubt I was in, that parenting is a demanding task.

The day was a sweet memory, when the doctor informed me that I was an expecting mother. A peace and tranquillity was all over me. An amalgamation of excitement, fear, insecurity all together were creating a turmoil in me which was inexpressible.

The special day when my angel was in my arms and on the other side a shy, submissive girl transformed into a mother -with a new soul in my arms. New motherhood catapulted me into caring, careful and a responsible being. The heavenly grace and the compassion flowing into me from heaven above.

But here I was wrong, to even think that my life has become a topsy -turvy now. The fact is that each member of the family has to contribute and play his or her part in bringing up the child. What the newborn needs is a congenial atmosphere for a balanced growth. The members of the family play a crucial role in order to shape the child's character and his well being. If the child is brought up in a joint family, he then easily adapts in the society or any organisation he is in the future. On the other hand, the parents can be the support system to guide the child. Keeping a protection shield along with nurturing and feeding him till he is not independent.

As I was going through one of Isha Sadguru's lectures, he has rightly says-

" To parent a child - a hundred percent commitment for the next twenty years, once he enters your life. If one starts living a conscious life, then the journey of parenthood would be less challenging".

So this myth should be broken that we have to parent a child. The fact is that the child only needs guidance and protection to live a healthy and happy life. Half of the job is done, if a conscious approach is practised on a daily basis.Parents have only to be aware of their own actions , thoughts and value systems.

Self-Realisation before child birth

The need of addressing underlying psychological issues-

After marriage, modern and sensible couples plan their family according to the physical and mental state of mind. They are fully aware of the appropriate time to prepare themselves for parenthood.

On the basis of my personal experience as a parent and a Parental Coach, my research has helped me to put forth some important points which the newly should keep in mind and to develop certain traits, before they enter the Parenthood.

The three nuggets which a couple needs to follow religiously are:

Patience-

Tolerance

Awareness

Lets understand these in detail-

***Patience-**

This is the most needed trait which is to be inculcated in the To-b e-Parents.Reason is that nothing is expected in Parenthood, which is challenging. But if we wait and watch it for a while and get into the root cause, things get far better than expected. It doesn't remain a struggle any more, instead it helps us to enjoy parenthood.

It is obvious that before the child is born, their own childhood is still hovering on the couples, as they are under the love and care of their own parents. Being restless, young , impatient and ignorant about parenthood, they need some value-time to internalise this. Get themselves educated by elders about their forthcoming responsibilities.

The child born to thoughtful and responsible parents grow into sensible citizens and on the other hand, children born to irresponsible and ignorant parents may become a burden to the society. So, what I thought before. So, the crux is that before going into parenthood, newly married couples should work upon their weaknesses. There are only a few which are needed to be worked upon before the journey of Parenthood begins. You are all set to enter into the phase of Parenthood.

Outcome- Helps the growing child to bond with the parents

***Tolerance-**

The second most important factor is being tolerant. One can start being tolerant of the behaviour of the children you are around with. As all children behave similarly, everybody is not tolerant towards them. The children need a different approach to deal with, as they are sensitive, idealistic and sharp.

It is essential to know how a baby grows and develops in pregnancy to understand the   importance of antenatal care for the health of the mother and baby.

After birth, a child will do whatever is needed to fulfil his physiological needs, which is a demanding task. The couple who has just entered into parenthood, should remember that this phase is not going to last for long. Enjoy the phase you will never regret it and these will remain sweet memories which are there with the blessed ones.

Outcome- Helps to form a deep spiritual connection with the child

***Awareness-**

1.My experience of childbirth has taught me an important lesson:

That awareness of your own body both physiologically and emotionally is very important for the expecting mother; The development of the baby in the uterus from conception to birth. The routine tests which are offered as part of antenatal care should be taken with utmost care

2. The expectant mother can stay healthy in pregnancy if she is at her conscious level to give birth to a healthy baby.

3. She remains attentive to both dietary and lifestyle advice.

4. The meditative and breathing processes to be worked upon. Appropriate counselling is needed for preparing her through the pregnancy period.

5. Stay happy and feel blessed because the Universe has chosen you to parent his creation on this earth.

Outcome- Mistakes can be avoided to some extent.

***Develop a good listening skill:**

Marriage is an arrangement in which two individuals work for a common purpose- to make a congenial atmosphere for a new soul to enter your world.

And the most important aspect of any relationship is communication and a healthy rapport among the family members. Right after marriage, if a couple seriously thinks about their family, they have to work upon themselves.

The basic need of this arrangement is to raise a family, with healthy children. A child is the sum total of people around him and his future lies in what the environment offers him to become in his future. So, the common thing which flows in all relationships to make it a congenial one is good listening skill.

When the two families come together, there will be differences of opinions but a good listening skill will save all odds. This is the most important skill needed for the parents to inculcate the same in their children.

A patient mindset is what is required for preparation towards parenthood. Sensible couples start training themselves patiently. For that they should practise this skill, in order to strengthen the bonding. In such an environment, the child develops a good listening skill. To develop this skill one , one needs to remain calm, which will help to grasp new ideas and information. This is the time when the couple should start inculcating this habit , listening to the elders and their experiences. This will help them to plan and prepare for a balanced parenthood.

Outcome- The child will be trained to keep calm in the face of challenges.

Caring for one's own Health-

Caring for one's health is a far-sighted thought.

My aim of mentioning these important points is not to overwhelm the readers but to make the journey of Parenthood a joyful one. It is the highest of happiness for the parents to watch their children grow into healthy and stable citizens of this planet.

My experiences as a daughter and a parent, has provided me certain insights, which I believe the younger generations should not repeat.

It is not a moral policing, but in a certain way, to avoid unnecessary complex health issues during conception and later in life.

Health is a major part of our lives. It is rightly said that a healthy mind resides in a healthy body. It includes avoiding Junk Food, which has never proved as healthy for anyone. So expecting parents should be more careful, as these days many complications arise from bad eating habits.

The couples should slowly move to Home-made foods and that to Satwik foods. There are many examples around us where we can observe the complications which the children are prone to. Diseases like obesity and others related to childbirth are common these days.

Firstly, the aim of starting to eat consciously and slowly becomes a Habit. When the child enters your life, then it would not be difficult to switch over to a diet plan prescribed by the doctor or elders in the family. It includes fresh fruits , vegetables, diary products, nuts and other supplements according to your body index.

Secondly, eating healthy will help the unborn child and the mother to be healthy.This can even save the hassles of other complications of the child birth. When the parents develop a lifestyle of eating healthy, they can live a disease free life. Thus, giving birth to a healthy child, securing the child's future.

Outcome- To nurture your child to live a healthy lifestyle, without much resistance.

BE RESPECTFUL
Will you listen to someone, who doesn't talk nicely to you? When we give respect to our children, it helps them radiate it back to you too.

Start working on your communication skills-

A good communication skill is a blessing in disguise. Many lives are affected, if one does not develop his/her communication skills. In our modern world, strenuous physical activities have taken a back seat. We should be grateful to technology, as now we have ample time to work on our soft skills- communication.

If parents know that they lack this trait in their personality. Then in that case, they can make this as their top priority and stay aware of how to improve these skills. There are various options in the market, such as online speaking courses,personality building, etc.

It is a well known fact that communication begins right at home. A child learns the mother tongue, pronunciation, tone of the language well before he interacts with the world outside his home or school. So, if the parents are not fluent with the language, there is nothing to worry about.

The way you talk and polite interaction with the child may do wonders. For that one has to become a role model for the child. Remember that each time you open your mouth in the presence of your child, he will listen and try to imitate you.

Don't get me wrong here. The point which I am laying stress upon is the way one communicates leads towards respect for others. It will not only help in inculcating good values in your child but also keep your home in peace and tranquillity in future.

Better the communication skills, the better will be the relationships among family and friends. Communication is the root cause of love and hatred in this world. Once you have worked upon yourself, it will then become very easy to pave a life for your child to take care of his relationships easily.

Outcome- Communication is a medium to express love and feel loved.

Disciplined life-

Our scriptures and Holy books are the easiest way to understand the importance of Discipline. All religions are based on DISCIPLINE.

So here each one of us knows the importance of DISCIPLINE but it takes a huge effort to stay in this zone. Each day has something new for all of us if we stay active and aware of it. In the same way, the child picks up all kinds of actions which elders or their parents are seen doing in their presence.

The mannerism, way of talking, style of walking ,even dressing up is observed by the child. The child not only observes you but also observes your behaviour with detailed precision. He tries to pick up the good habits as he does the bad habits. SO the role of the parent is of utmost importance, as they are the first teachers of the child. The sad part of it is that they themselves do not acknowledge it, and keep blaming the society and the environment.

So the role of the parent should not be taken casually. Nothing is to be worried about, but a conscious parenting is needed. Kids are watching you, so just remain attentive, at least, in front of your children.

Outcome- Your Kids are your own mirror- image.

There are common ways to stay rooted and rewind yourself, for the sake of your child's betterment. Do not get overwhelmed, to worry about these things, most of which are ingrained in your behaviour. Have to be a little conscious about yourself, as a result ,your parenting journey will be at ease.

In addition-

Take care of your hygiene.

Plan out an exercise regime.

Get a personalised diet plan from a certified Nutritionist

Morning walk with your spouse will do wonders in your relationship too.

Sufficient sleep.

All this will seem to be so easy and enjoyable, that you will discover a new YOU, which will also help you to be more confident at your work-place and also in your relationships. Hence, we can conclude with-

' A Happy Parent will nurture happy children'

Summary of the Chapter-1

1. Prepare well to become a better Parent.

2. Self-realisation about one's action.

3. Address your own Psychological issues.

4. Have Patience

5. Practical Tolerance

6. Develop Awareness

7. Treat yourself well and heal your inner child

8. Develop a good listening skill.

9. Be caring for one's own Health

10. Work on your Communication skills.

11. Inculcate a Disciplined Lifestyle.

Chapter 2
Urgent Need to Learn Behavioural Parenting

What is Behaviour ?

Behaviour is anything that can be seen, observed or measured as greeting someone, helping someone. It involves verbal as well as non-verbal behaviour.

Ideas for Parents

Q.1. How do we train the children to become independent?

- Set a right example for your child

- Trust your child

- Let the child learn according to his appropriate age

- Let him make his own decisions

e.g.ask him which coloured shirt he wants to wear.

- Create opportunities for your child.

e.g.Let him decide what should be made for lunch etc.

- Ask more questions, instead of providing suggestions

- Do not criticise your child or compare him with others

Q.2. Why are the children shy and lack confidence?

Ans. It is to be understood that a shy child can be confident.

The child may be quiet and trying to learn certain things on   his own. Or maybe hiding some grudge or being unable to speak   clearly because of some sort of fear.

Q.3. How can we train our children about time-management?

Ans To start training your child for time-management-

- Develop mind-management- Training the child to make a schedule or time-table for his day , week and months.

- In the first place, parents should schedule his picnics, excursions, tracking or few other exciting activities.

- Shift in mental perspectives- train your child to make a decision to prioritise his actions. Let your child decide which is the most important for him and which is less.

- Identify the skills of your child- It is important for the parents to make an effort so that he does all his activities with passion and concentration.

Q. 4. How can the parents train their children to communicate well ?

Ans- To encourage your children to speak-

- Listen to them with patience and sincerity

- Maintain eye-contact with your child.

- Try to share your thoughts with the child

- They learn by imitation. Some may learn to communicate faster while others are slow.

- Use of decent vocabulary mainly while one is talking while children are around.

- Lastly do not pressurise them to talk if they do not want to.

- If you feel, you can consult a good speech therapist if the child is slow- learner.

Q.5. My elder son is slow and shy as compared to the younger one. I am worried about him. What can I do to help him?

Ans- In the first place, labelling your child is the most harmful aspect of parenting. Parents are Supreme for the child, any word uttered by them becomes a truth for the child, he blindly follows them. So, calling your child slow, lethargic, angry, fearful, shy etc. puts a lot of burden on the child as his brain is still developing.

Here I recollect, the famous episode in little Edison's life,

Whenever you have two or three kids, in this case we are the most careful parents only for the eldest one. He is checked by both the parents too closely, as both the parents are young and energetic. In addition to it they take this new role too seriously. The first child is looked after by both parents. As a result the child's own personality remains in a recessive mode.

As soon as the second child enters the family, the parents' complete focus shifts towards the new one as it is the need of the hour. But somewhere the elder one gets into his shell as he is not provided with the same attention by the parents now. The worst happens when parents start comparing both the children- this has a negative impact on the child. The result is that the elder one does not put much effort to prove himself, so gets into his safe zone.

Appreciation - Look for opportunities to appreciate the child. Praise is a short term tool. Praise the child for his behaviour but not the child.

1.Focus on the child's action OR behaviour, only those actions which we want the child to learn.

2. Appreciate with energy

3. No false praise and not for everything

4. Praise the child immediately after his accepted behaviour.

5. Focus on the process , not on the child.

6. Growth mindset

There is Behaviour Modification therapy, which involves taking an undesirable or unwanted behaviour and replacing that with a more desirable and more acceptable behaviour.

It involves-

Skill training

Cognitive Training

Brain training

Social Training

Emotional training

And all of these targets are achieved with practising it in play, involving them in games, activities, which in turn helps in child to increase

- Sitting tolerance

- Attention

- Cognitive ability

- To remove the problematic behaviour

There are various Specialists in the professional world:

Early Interventionist

Paediatric Physiotherapist

Speech Language Pathologist

Special educator

Occupational Therapist

Behaviour Therapist

We should look around us and seek assistance whenever you feel your child needs at the correct time. It is to involve your child too. Make him understand about its importance in this way he will feel more confident and boldly try to help you.

__Summary of the Chapter-2__

Urgent need to learn Behavioural Parenting

1. Behaviour is anything that can be seen or observed. It includes

<u>Verbal</u>- The way we talk to others.

<u>Non-Verbal</u>- The way we talk or deal with others at emotional or mental level.

Behavioural Parenting is to prepare your child for life.

1. Trust your child

2. Create opportunities for him

3. Train him to take his own decisions

4. Do not compare him with others.

5. Ask Questions rather than providing suggestions

6. Inculcate the importance of time-management.

7. Help the child to communicate well.

8. Be a good listener for your child.

9. Appreciation is needed but it should be genuine and specific. It will make him proud.

Chapter 3
Responsible Parenting

What I have observed, that Parenting itself is a term related to responsibility. So coining such a term is pointless, when it comes to parenting.

This term is adopted directly from Latin *parentem*, from PIE root *pere- "to produce, bring forth".

BE READY FOR A TANTRUM
Whenever you say No to your child, just be prepared that there will be a tantrum to convince you somehow. Even if we say No politely, they will cry to see if you will give it to them or not.

Important Role of Parents

What if the parents play their part with responsibility and concern-keeping in view the far-fetched consequences. If they play their part with utmost consciousness, their child will be a contributor in making this world a better place.

After going through various histories and researches, I have come to a conclusion that the root cause of a better as well as worse society depends upon responsible parenting only. If we dig deeper into the larger scenario of the world, it is the parents who shape the future of their child and the society on the whole.

There are best examples of Responsible Parenting in our world.

1. **<u>Thomas Edison's Mother, brought new light in the Parent-Child Relationship</u>**

Most loved and appreciated is the Parenting style of Thomas Edison's mother. This is a well-known story of the responsible parenting-

One day Thomas Edison came home and gave a paper to his mother. HE TOLD HER, "My teacher gave this paper to me and told me to only give it to my mother".

His mother's eyes were tearful as she read the letter out loud to her child: Your son is a genius. This school is too small for him and doesn't have enough good teachers for training him. Please teach him yourself.

After many many years, after Edison's mother died and he was one of the greatest inventors of the century, one day he was looking through old family things. Suddenly he saw a folded piece of paper in the corner of a desk drawer. He took it and opened it up. On the paper was written: Your son is addled(mentally ill). We won't let him come to the school anymore.

Edison cried for hours and then he wrote in his diary: Thomas ALVA Edison was an addled child, by a hero mother, became the genius of the century".

Though this story is a famous one. Even so, I could not stop myself from writing it here- for my readers. So that they get a direct message which fulfils my mission to write this book.

It is never too late to learn and unlearn certain things, when it comes to parenting. The most fond memories of a person is his childhood. So, as parents, let us take a pledge to provide a wonderful experience of childhood for your angel.

2. Shivaji, the great-

He was one of the most intelligent and brave personalities of historical India. He too was influenced by his mother. She inspired him to be brave and smart from early childhood. She inculcated the leadership qualities in him. Inspired him with stories and tales of brave personalities. Her thoughtfulness later made him one of the most effective rulers, who fought the Mughals bravely. Till today, many of the combat wars today are inspired by his war strategies. He was an effective planner and a mentally-strong personality.

<u>Reason</u>- The childhood stage has a short span. Once the child enters into teens, it becomes more challenging for the parents to rectify the unwanted behaviour.

Some common **mistakes** which parents make due to ignorance or in a spurt of emotional burst.

- **Comparisons**

According to researchers in the field of Psychology, parents are in the habit of comparing their children. Sometimes with their friends and even with their siblings. It is not intentionally or to hurt their child, but only because of human nature. If we are aware of this human character, we realise that each one of us is behaving in such a manner. Then why is the parent always made to feel guilty for a common human trait? This is a human nature which the child psychologist and the counsellors keep highlighting, whenever the issue of Parenting is dealt with.

The reason is obvious, that this is the soft spot for the child, which lingers on in his memories even in the adult stage of life.

I have come across many parents, in my Coaching and counselling journey, who themselves are the victim of unforgettable childhood ex-periences. They can recall each incident with minute detail- as it has left a deep mark on his emotions.

The sad part of parenting is that they never have such intentions- but even then children take them wrong.

So, here we have to carefully assist the parents and help them by continuous counselling and one to one sessions.

- **Preach before practising-**

This is the most common mistake which the majority of parents make due to ignorance. We all have heard this phrase:

'To err is human'. So though as parents we do not follow what we would like our children to practise. Firstly, the reason is again love for the child and secondly, the consequences which they have faced should not be suffered by their kids.But it doesn't work that way. Children hardly listen or even understand the spoken message. Whatever they observe, becomes the truth. This is the reason why Conscious Parenting is promulgated.

For example - The children who hit others, usually have a role model for aggression at home.

As a parent, it becomes our Moral duty towards our kids, to model our traits, which we expect them to learn.

For example-

To remain humane is the basis of any kind of relationship.

Respect for elders and fellow beings.

Honesty in our actions.

Kindness towards the needy.

- **Lack of Tolerance**- The most important trait is that of tolerance which is needed to be a part of one's character. This is the most important because it lets many people stay in a congenial environment ,which is to be inculcated during childhood.

'To lose Patience, is to lose a battle'

-- Mahatma Gandhi

There is no rocket science to become a calm and patient parent. But most of the time, they lose their temper resulting in dire consequences.

Childhood is the most vulnerable stage of life. The child may face these recessive symptoms- which the parents may observe in the later stages of life. These are as listed below:

1. Continuous headaches, thumb-sucking, mild fever, allergies and many other psychological issues. These may remain recessive in a few individuals.

2. Major health issues like Cancer, kidney stones, thyroid, Blood pressure etc.in the later stages of life.

Hence, Modern Child Psychology has given rise to a support system for the parents to educate themselves. The parents ought to seek help and guidance in the initial days of parenthood. Both the child and the parents would be saved from wasting time in sorting out issues on their own.

There is a wonderful Quote by Samuel. R. Delemy,

"We try to bring up our children, so that they are protected from the world's evil, only to find, we have raised a pack of innocents, who seem to be,about to stumble into, at every turn, just for sheer stupidity".

Does punishment work ?

When I was punished, my parents often had this statement - "You are older than your sister, should have taken care or behaved sensibly". I could not understand, even the meaning of behaving sensibly in the first place and what was my mistake for which I was getting scolded. I do however remember the anger I felt towards my parents. I can only recall from -how I had developed the habit of pinching my siblings, in order to vent out my frustration for being scolded unnecessarily. And I even had invented my own ways to get appreciation from my parents, that even led to thinking ways, how to impress them,so that I also could receive appreciation from them. This was a huge distraction from my studies. I even could not realise how much time I had wasted from my study schedule.

1. This same pattern I could identify in my students also. Where parents told me that our child studies for long hours, but they were worried that they were not able to score good in their exams.

2. I came across many students in my teaching career, who were serious about their studies but their show up rate was less. Some of them were so concerned about their academics that they even were afraid to participate in co -curricular activities.

3. As a result the happiness quotient of such children is so low that they feel stressed at the basic level. Resulting in a sad state of mind or depression.

4. Many of them were sportsmen, but could not pursue their passion. Again the reason was lack of concentration. These children had talents but could not outshine. Such children start developing a sense of insecurity and they themselves are not aware of it.

- Shy

- Submissive

- Docile

- Lack confidence

- Insecure

- No self-belief

- Lack of concentration

My observation and experience of almost 15 years with children of all age groups, that the environment and the mindset play a vital role in a human being's life.

In some cases, even a single family member or friend makes him feel good about his qualities and talents, making a huge difference in his perception of life. The child ONLY needs a patient listening and understanding,

The rest of the matters are well-handled by the child himself, he knows well what he is expected to work upon.

1. Hormonal Imbalance: The main reason here is that he is in a stage where hormonal imbalance occurs. He is over-emotional and can react to even the minor of the incidents in his life. The turmoil disturbs him and prevents him from thinking in a logical manner.

2. Hypersensitivity: Preteens get disturbed when they are treated as kids. They are trying to imitate the grown ups and hate to be dictated as kids. The reason is that they are observing everybody around them. Whatever has been taught to them, proves to be unreal. He starts questioning his parents and gets a positive response which satisfies his thinking mind. In such cases, the most of the clarity he receives from his parents, at home itself. But what about those children who live with an authoritative or a permissive parent. He is sure to get his answers from the outside world.

3. Approach of the Parents: The approach should be a balanced one. The children are continuously looking forward to their Parents for appreciation. Here, the parents need to practise- 'to appreciate appropriately'.

In most of the families, parents do not appreciate the child for any task of his, fearing that the child will get spoiled or will not inculcate discipline. On the other hand, some families are so lenient towards the child, that he grows up with zero- tolerance towards criticism. So, a parent needs to analyse the situation with a far-sighted approach. How much appreciation the child is supposed to get and how much he needs to be kept in check - is the duty of the parent so that the child grows with a balanced mindset.

Pearson's Law: " When performance is measured, performance improves.

When performance is measured and reported back, the rate of improvement accelerates".

<u>Summary Of Chapter-3</u>

Responsible Parenting:

1. **Important Role of Parenting in Child's Life**- A balanced approach is all what the child needs when he is growing. Nothing much.

2. **Create Leaders**- Child is not to be dictated but to be guided, so that he is able to lead an independent and a responsible life.

3. **Parenting Flaws-**

- Comparisons between siblings may lead to sibling rivalry.

- Preaching before practising

- Lack of tolerance towards children

- Unconscious use of language

- Snubbing the child

- Apply a short term -approach

- Play with the child's- psychology without understanding

1. **Punishment - is it important?**

It is a controversial aspect of parenting. Some promulgate it , while others may understand it as discouraging.

Again this aspect of Parenting needs a lot of debate and it needs a complete mindshift. The reason is that it is challenging as sometimes it boomerangs, if not handled with care.

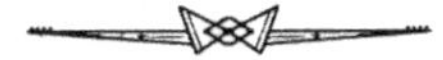

Chapter 4

Shaping The Emotional Personality

As a parent I have observed this fact in a hard way. If the surrounding is not conducive for the parent, it is in an auto-mode that we try to adjust the child accordingly. To bring up a child, it is not something we can take lightly. There is hardly any clarity to how and what should be the perfect method to raise a child. As, raising a child is not a temporary job, but a deal for at least 20 years. It is because we are not preparing him for a day or a year, but for a life. It is the most responsible and methodical job assigned by the Almighty, to make this earth a place with sensible citizens.

Here the parent gets overwhelmed, Instead of moving patiently towards his goal, he is looking forward to quick results. Here we all parents commit a huge mistake.

It is rightly said that, 'The work done in a rush is a devil's work'.

Here the Behavioural Therapy comes to play.

Functional Behaviour Analysis: Every behaviour serves a function, the child's behaviour needs attention. Three things are essential:

1. Define the problem behaviour clearly- HOW the behaviour sounds or looks like?

2. What child is getting from doing that behaviour in that way?

3. What is the child avoiding by doing that behaviour?

4. What the child is doing before the behaviour is happening- is called as Antecedent

5. And what is happening after the behaviour - Consequence

Parenting is a blessing in disguise. It is only bestowed upon a person, to look after the child but also, to inculcate patience. It is time that the individual calms down his nerves. The only mindset he should be, that he is constantly being observed and looked upon.

Parenting is not an humongous task, as we have projected it. It is only one's own mirror image, in a child. Only we can go for a better version of ourselves if we work carefully towards it.

When a child is born, the parent naturally enters the state of love and care. He or she gets into an auto mode of protection of the little one.

The same happened with me too. The most lethargic and carefree girl instantly became **the most responsible** being on this earth. Turned into Conscious Parent, even though most of the time things were out of control. Unknowingly, my frustrations tumbled on my children. I was in a mindset that if I share my challenges and hurdles with my children, they may learn some life lessons. Suffered with self - doubt, each time a new problem raised its head. The mistake which I was ignorant of was-committing to feel that I am being heard. But on the contrary, they were supposed to be heard. I had been, throughout my parenting journey, throwing my emotional baggage on the growing children. Thus making their journey more saddening. This realisation came to me, when their academics were affected . Here lies the crux when we ourselves end up pulling our child back, instead of bringing joy during their childhood. Today they are the most sensible beings, but I could understand this the day I realised that they were growing fast.

Positive Parenting:

Nuggets which I would like to share with my readers are as follows

1. Children are adorable: Take it easy, each day carefully. The way the artist shapes his piece of Art. The effort we put in our child, will reap its outcomes.

2. Appreciating the child: This is the most important aspect of Parenting, which is mostly neglected. Parents are of the opinion that appreciating the child will pamper him. But this is absolutely a wrong notion.

3. Perception: The child is growing at his own pace. Each day comes with a new experience for him, as he is into a learning phase. The way he perceives things is entirely different from that of the elders.

For example, playing with the child for some time with the child.

4. Confidence- If the child does not take a stand for his rights or remains submissive, depicts that the parents mindset has influenced their thought process. Their can be two factors-

Either the personality of the parents has overshadowed his or a new one is evolving.

5. Independent- If we are overprotective, it is equivalent to clipping his wings to fly. In such cases do not expect your child to use his own brains. The reason is your grooming, in such a manner, that he fails to decide for himself.

His perception is not on the same plane, confusing him to a larger extent.

6. Way of conversing- 'Watch your tongue'- This may appear strange to some parents, but this has a huge role to play with his emotions. How

we talk to our child matters a lot, which may have a lifelong influence on the child's innate personality. As a highly emotional parent, I have been committing this blunder throughout my Parenting journey.

Adding to the child's agony, the parents and the teachers are equally responsible for his fearful personality which hinders his mental growth.

1. Montessori Method: My own experiences in Montessori schools has provided me an insight that it is to some extent, tailor made for the child. In this kind of methodology, the child is helped to grow, in a way that he doesn't get overwhelmed. Reason being that it is at his own pace.

2. Anxiety issues and Childish overthinking: In my opinion, daydreaming and overthinking are the main areas where the child gets stuck. So, continuous conversations with the child are the most important. During childhood, if the anxiety issues are taken care of, it helps the child to ponder over his self growth and intelligence. His energies are channelised-resulting into a confident personality.

3. Language learning: Parents and the elders lay lots of stress on Language learning. But how many of us react in the manner that the child doesn't get overwhelmed. Fear has prevented him from expressing, but he is capable of scanning your intentions. He has already painted a fearful picture of the others just because of those he comes in contact with. As a result his neurons have already been conditioned in a way that anyone talking loud and rude becomes scary for the child.

4. Impact of Negative Parenting: The child's mind receives reassurance about being fearful of everything that comes in the way. This may trigger

other consequences like stammering, nail-biting, bed-wetting, continuous headaches, thumb-sucking, mild fever, allergies and many other psychological issues. These may remain recessive in a few individuals. Thus leading to greater health issues like Cancer, kidney stones, thyroid, Blood pressure etc.in the later stages of life.

Hence, Modern Child Psychology has given rise to a support system for the parents to educate themselves. The parents ought to seek help and guidance in the initial days of parenthood. Both the child and the parents would be saved from wasting time in sorting out issues on their own.

There is a wonderful Quote by Samuel. R. Delemy,

"We try to bring up our children, so that they are protected from the world 's evil, only to find , we have raised a pack of innocents, who seem to be,about to stumble into, at every turn, just for sheer stupidity".

Chapter 5
Relationships

My best friend had suggested a book which I should read. It was **'Dusk Night Dawn'**- by Anne Lammote. Being a Parent myself I could resonate with the emotion connected with it.

The author has mentioned her parents in a dark shade. I felt that she was holding a grudge against them. Frankly, she has described her mother both as a terrorist and a child. She is not mincing her words to describe her father as a womaniser. This description about her parents, during her adult life, truly reverberates to many of us, at a conscious level. The tragic aspect is that she has undergone these experiences during her childhood. Are you on the same plane, which makes me present this story.

Lesson learnt from this true experience -

The parents who are the solid pillars of the child, should take an oath-

"Come what may; whether marital or financial issues, should be resolved keeping in view their child's future. So that the child's core personality should not be influenced due to the parents".

There is a famous idiom to coin the differences between the parents- **'To bury the hatchet'**-

This is an essential element, by which you can work together for your child's betterment. This is not what is being promulgated by someone, but it is the best decision which both the parents should make. It is in a moment that two adults try to escape from carrying the burden of relationship. In a sense, they act in a self-centred manner.

It is a matter of positive thinking, if both come on a common consent- the child. The only aim is to save the child from untoward consequences which he might face in the presence of any one of the parents. This is such a decision which is not a comfortable one for the couple but they may thank each other when they observe their child growing in a balanced way.

There are many examples in our society because of the wrong decisions of the parents.

BE CALM
Just remain calm and composed even if there is screaming and shouting by your child when you said No. By loosing your temper you will just add fuel to the fire.

- <u>**Confidence**</u>- Confidence is the might and right of the child which helps him to live a complete life.

Once the confidence level of the child drops, it then costs him a lot, hence forcing him into insecurity of all kinds.

For example- Most of the cases seen in the society where the children get into consuming drugs and other bad habits. The reason is that they find it difficult to be heard.

The lack of achievement is the result and that may again lead to other complicacies like self-pity, suicidal thoughts, depression etc.

I came into contact with a young student of mine. He used to consume liquor, whenever he got the opportunity. On having a discussion with him regarding this Habit, it was revealed that both the parents were into this bad habit. Parents being overbusy, in their business,could not spend time together as well as the children.As a result both the parents, engrossed in their own world, did not bother much about their children.

Consequences were obvious that the children felt neglected and also felt no harm in consuming liqour. It is normal for the child as he has been conditioned in such an environment.

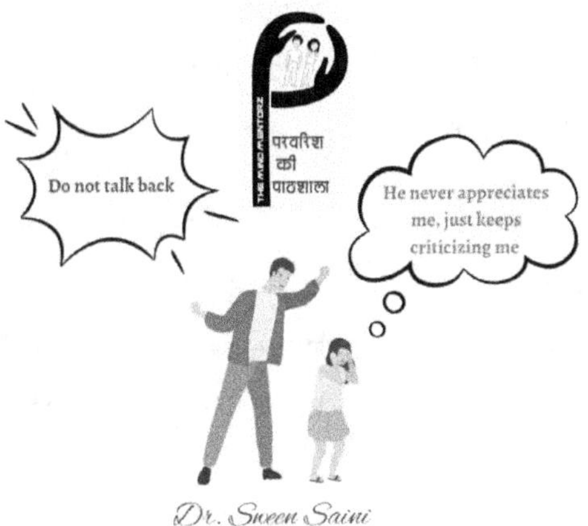

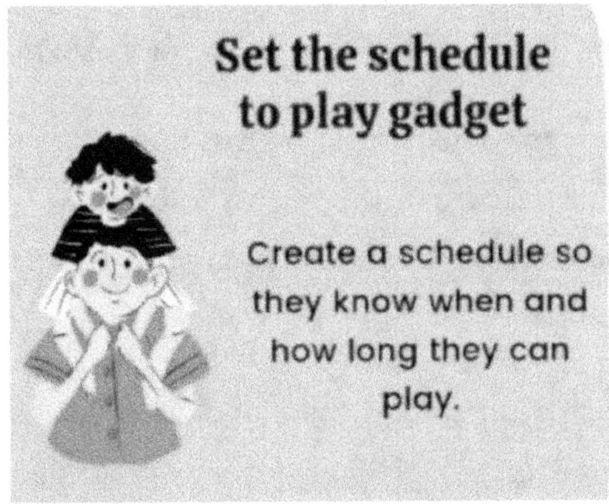

- **<u>Relationships</u>** - A distorted implication of relationship,

For Instance- I had come across an interview of a famous cricketer. When he was asked about his marriage plans; his reply was that he never believed in the arrangement of marriage, just because his parents had a disturbed relationship. He had an insecurity related to marriage and commitment towards a permanent relationship.

So, I think my readers could get an idea, how the child develops a distorted concept about marriage, which seems to be the most awaited enduring arrangement in one's life.

Marriage- It is the beginning of the family and a life-long commitment. Then what on earth, permits the parents to disturb the whole arrangement for the child. Alongwith growing selflessly towards a common goal of nurturing the child. For a child both the parents have separate roles to play and to be "on the same page".

According to our Scriptures, marriage is not a man-made law. It is the arrangement of the Power above. That is why, it is believed that - the reason and feeling in man and woman should be balanced.

Emotional Support- The parents engross themselves to earn wealth, that they miss out the precious moments to be spent with their little angels. When these angels grow up, then the vicious cycle again starts.

The child's priority is not economic support but it is more of an emotional one. At such a juncture of childhood, when he is vulnerable and needs full support in growing happily towards adulthood.

Why such atrocities towards our own children? Are they at fault? Or their fault is that they are born to careless parents.

What about their emotional and psychological hampering of their personality?

<u>**Parental support-**</u>

Without parental support, the child will have to struggle a lot even for his basic needs.

On a large scale, the education world is moving towards modifications and changes in methodology and approach. It is leading the world towards a child-centred arrangement. This is excellent, but do you think any of these methods would be a success-

Now the Parents have to work upon themselves, in order to make this kind of education system a success.

The society which is child-centred is successful to an extent. It can be considered as a happy one.

It is a well known fact that the childhood experience is the most impressionable one. The learning and behaviour is by imitating the elders. It's not only behaving but also acting in a manner in which to be receptive about. Like for example- the family which prays together and eats together makes their children feel warmth of belongingness beyond words.

Modern parents also go to the extent of playing with them. That feeling is an awesome one, during which his sweet memories get imprinted. I think game time is the most crucial one. It helps the parent to connect deeply with the child and understand his psychology more deeply.

This is easy if the parents and people around always make sure that the child's mind should be trained for a Logical thinking. In this way, he will be learning new things in his own unique way rather than get in a biassed state of mind. The synonym of biassed is prejudice or predilection. According to dictionary,

"It implies an unreasoned and unfair distortion of Judgement in favour or against a person or thing".

Parents ignorantly or intentionally, hamper their child's COGNITIVE THINKING.

Here is when this type of thinking may take the shape of Cognitive biases. It can negatively impact our minds to think critically and may hamper our decision- making.

Now what the parents are habitual of is validating the actions and attitudes. In this way, by confirming evidence, kids are made to feel good.

My research about this aspect, helps me to conclude that for some parents and the children, following this method keeps them in a comfort zone.

First Reason: This method proves to be easier and faster.

I have also come across those parents who follow the Scientific Path of answering each and every question of the child. Though this is too exhausting, only if you take it as a job. But it is a blessing to wait for the child for his queries.

I would like to remind the parents that this arrangement will not last for long. You will be proud of spending qualitative time with your child in the later stage of life.

Second Reason: Your child will develop Cognitive thinking in almost all areas of his life. His decision-making will be based on logic. What more would a parent wish for, if his child has the capability to work with numbers and to reason well.

Summary Of Chapter-5

Relationship is based on following factors-

1. Self Confidence is the key for a child to live happily in future.

2. Sanctity of Marriage, needs to be examplified for the children. Onus lies on the parents and they have got to make sure of it, that the child respects this relationship.

3. Emotional support, if provided by the parents goes a long way.

4. Parental support, is what makes the child respect and have faith in humanity.

5. Cognitive thinking, helps the child in decision- making. Conscious Parenting plays an important role to develop this approach.

6. Two important reasons-

(I) Scientific Path

(2) Logical Thinking

Chapter 6
Logical Thinking

"At the end of the day, the most overwhelming key to a child's success is the positive involvement of the parents". – Jane D.Hull

Logical Thinking plays a vital role in each one of our lives. A skill which all the parents wish their child to develop. The critical thinking skills when practised in logic can also be applied in sound decision-making.

It is observed that parents encourage their children to learn and Practise Logical thinking. For this trait to be inculcated in the child, they have to pay a close attention to details of the child's experiences.

Logic - means a science of reasoning.

Logical thinking is the ability to analyse a situation in order to come to a rational conclusion. If a child is trained to make a distinction between right and wrong, it will have a huge impact on his daily life and his happiness quotient.

- Positive effects of logical thinking skills on children:

- They are successful at school.

- Helps the child to establish cause and effect relations.

Brain Anatomy

To understand the Human brain, we have to go deeper into the functioning of our central nervous system or CNS.

The human brain and spinal cord are the two important organs which constitute the CNS.

The brain is a complex organ that controls thought, memory, emotion, feel, touch, motor skills, vision , breathing, hunger, and regulates the temperature of the body.

The cerebrum(front of the brain) comprises of-

- Grey matter(cerebral cortex)

- White matter at its centre.

Functions of cerebrum-

1. Initiates and coordinates movement

2. Regulates temperature

Other areas of the cerebrum-

1. Enables speech

2. Judgement

3. Problem solving

4. Thinking and reasoning

5. Emotions and Learning

Brain Development in early childhood

It is scientifically proven that a child's brain develops from birth to age 5, more than any other time in life.

The child's brain develops according to the experiences he has faced in the first few years of life. The way his brain develops in the early stages has a great impact on the child's mental development. His ability to learn in school and his overall success in life depends on his early brain development.

It is a proven fact that

- The brain of a newborn is about a quarter of the size of an average adult brain.

- It doubles in size in the first year.

- It grows to about 80% of adult size by age 3.

- 90% -nearly full grown-by age 5.

The child is born with all the brain cells(neurons) but it's the connections between these cells that really make the brain work. The early childhood years are crucial for making these connections.

Neural Connections- (<u>SYNAPSES</u>)- Approx.one million new Neural connections are made every second, during childhood ,more than any other time in life.

Different areas of the brain are responsible for different abilities-

- Movement

- Language

- emotion

Each child develops into a unique personality with the help of the following -

- **<u>Quality of care</u>**- The relationships which the child experiences with the adults, has a huge impact on their brain development. It is the parents and family at home. Later they come in contact with child caregivers, teachers and other members of the community.

- **<u>Interaction</u>**- Parents and caregivers who provide care and attention, respond and interact with their child are working towards building his brain.

- **<u>Stimulation</u>**- In order to stimulate his brain towards learning NEW SKILLS, it is important to talk, sing, read and play with young children from the day they are born, for providing opportunities to explore their physical world.

The connections are formed in these early years which are needed for many important abilities like-

(a)Motivation

(b)Self-regulation

(c)Problem-solving

(d)Communication

Independent child-

Every parent's dream is having an Independent child, but how many of us are really putting efforts to fulfil this dream.

"Don't handicap your children by making their lives easy".

- *Robert A. Heinlein*

If your children are independent, you have provided them with the belief that they are competent and capable of and capable of taking care of themselves.

Jim Taylor- in one of his blogs, has defined the dependent ones as Contingent children.

- Need incentive from others

- Look for happiness around.

- Lack of own Inspiration

- Depend on their parents for decision-making

In his research he has identified five types of contingent children, depending on their temperament and their parents.

<u>Pleasers</u>- I grew up as a pleaser myself and was perceived as an ideal child. The reason was that I always craved for parents' love and appreciation. The outcome was that I always felt resentful with sadness and lack of confidence. Actually I could not be me in a true sense.

The lack of confidence results in the children who get conditioned in such a manner. The muscle needed to be joyful in all odds stays recessive in the inner self. Such children are more likely to get into depression mode easily, as they are not self- motivated.

Now the question arises how we can nurture a child to become independent.

1. Reading

<u>Reading</u> helps to expand the imagination in the children. Especially fiction is a work out for your imagination. Emotion , feeling , memories and excitement creates a fictional world in the pages of a book.

The *neocortex* and *thalamus* are responsible for controlling the brain's imagination.

*They learn new things.

*increase the vocabulary.

*encourages empathy.

*strengthens the writing ability of the child.

*to increase his vocabulary.

*Develops Communication skills.

*increase focus and memory.

2 . Connect with your child

To discipline the child, <u>connection</u> is the most important aspect. The pattern of thinking becomes subtle and logical.

If you want your child to develop confidence in him , start connecting with him. It is not that difficult to develop this kind of connectivity as he also is craving for winning your trust. When he feels so, then the magic begins in your relationship.

As a consequence of trust, your child's willingness to accept your suggestions and friendly advice, may lessen the constraints of a relationship. In this way, the child feels free to share anything with parents.

3. Engage with them

This is the reason why I have started my book, with the pre -task a parent needs to work on i.e. that's their own personality.

The most important of the traits a parent has is to develop their upper brain and stay calm and balanced. It includes the rational, logical and empathetic aspect.

If the parent engages with his child, a healthy conversation is initiated. As a result, he is able to ask the right kind of questions and helps the child to engage his upper brain.

We all know that the child mirrors the same behaviour and in this way the parents can avoid anger and getting triggered by the child.

1. Give them age appropriate choices-

As a mother, I gave my children choices like which game to play or which food they would like to have. It isn't here that the parent has to follow whatever the child says but choose between any two options.

Outcome- It helps the child to get involved in the process.

1. Allow the child to Imagine

Experts at Vanderbilt University studied the brain to learn about imagination. By using MRI machines, it was revealed that imagination exercises many parts of the brain.

A child has a world of imagination moving with him. Allow him to imagine , do not mock or snub him for doing so.

I can relate to this accurately because my daughter imitated her teachers in the same way as if students were in front of her. Could imagine 10 pieces of bricks a s10 students of her class. Scolded them in the same way as her teacher did in the school. It was such fun for me to see her.

In the same way, my son when he was a toddler imagined driving a truck which he had seen in a movie. He imagined driving a motor bike with so much precision that even asked me to sit behind his bike to walk a stretch of a distance when we had to walk to a place.

Outcome- Experiments prove that pretending allows children to explore their own feelings and emotions.

4. Consistency-

Parents need to maintain consistency in:

Communication

Affection

Materialistic needs

Emotional needs

Discipline Methods

Outcome-

- Child feels safe and secure.

- He learns to trust the parents.

- Healthy routines can be maintained

Lack of consistency may lead the child-

1. To develop unhealthy routines

2. Will find hard to trust the environment

3. Unsafe and insecure

4. To develop manipulative approach

5. Keeps them confused.

<u>Tip for the Parent</u>- Listen to your child without any reaction or face expression. Think, ponder over it and give your suggestion later.

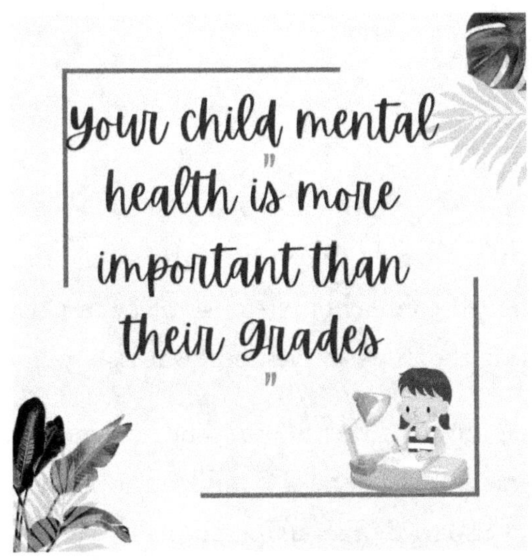

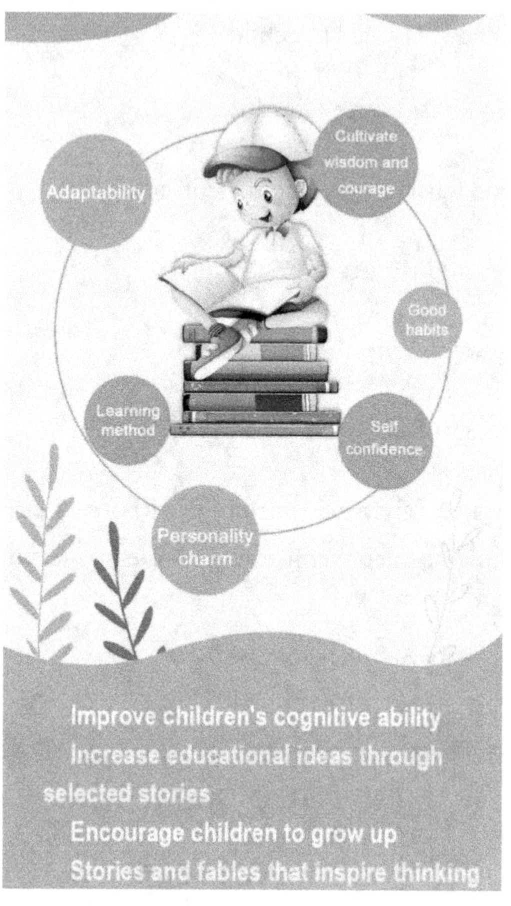

Almost every parent would dream- that their child develops into an independent and self-confident individual. Make sure that your child is able to do his daily chores or simplest of the tasks.

I would encourage my daughter to have food on her own once or twice. It helped her gradually to become confident not only to develop her eating habits but also tried other simple chores.

This helped her during kindergarten days also, she could complete her school task with confidence. She was the only student in her class who helped her teachers to take care of other students. Today I can feel that the leadership Qualities in her are the result of the early learnings.

The simple ways to encourage independence in your child-

1. Allow them to pick their own clothes from the cupboard.

2. Toilet habits to be developed as early as possible.

3. Help them to keep their toys at place after playing.

4. To fold their clothes.

5. To train the child to have his food independently.

6. Healthy eating to be encouraged with the help of appreciation.

There are some Proven Fun Ways to teach Logic to children-

Logic Puzzles- These are nowadays also a part of the school curriculum. e.g.

Syllogisms

Cryptograms

Arithmetic Puzzles

Chess Puzzles and many others.

Board Games- There are a number of easy Board Games,   which helps the children to develop a logical mindset. E.g.

The children can be given some popular games like Monopoly, Chutes & Ladders or Memory and many others.

E.g. Ludo and Carrom Board were the indoor games which children of our age have been playing during childhood. These were the games which kept them busy at home and the complete family played together at times. This was a time for me to communicate and spend some lighter moments with my parents. And I was anxiously waiting for this time in the evenings and these are those moments which have been added as one of the sweet childhood memories. Today we can see these because of technology, these games have been revived in mobiles also.

Brain training games-

SUDOKU

This is a brain challenging Number Placement game played on a 9x9 sudoku board. The sudoku board is broken down into nine 3x3 squares. It is a game in which the player has to analyse the grids and fill in the number. It is completely based on logic and relies on short term memory.

As a child, I was the first to fill the sudoku in the morning newspaper and felt proud to complete it . These days we can find it in our mobiles.

Crosswords

This was also one of my favourite childhood games. This was the game which my father also spared some time to play with me. It was introduced by him in order to increase my English vocabulary.

There are many other established brain training and mental fitness games which are backed by science. Some are listed as below:

Lumosity, Elevate, Peak, Happy Neuron, Braingle, Queendom, Wordle, Brain Age Concentration Training etc.

<u>Summary of Chapter-6</u>

1. Logical Reasoning is an ability to analyze a situation.

2. Brain anatomy

3. Neural connections.

4. Preparing an independent child.

*Reading

*Connecting with your child

*Engaging with them

*Giving them age-appropriate choices.

* Providing opportunities to imagine.

* Consistency in communication, feelings, emotional needs and discipline.

* Tips for the Parents

Chapter 7
Communication

"The way we treat our children directly impacts what they believe about themselves". - Ariadne Brill

*T*he first connection we make with our child is through communication- verbal as well as non-verbal. My experience has taught me that it is non-verbal in the beginning. The parent needs to be smart enough to understand what his child is imbibing. Being a parent is also a learning phase for an individual. The behaviour or action which didn't go well, should be looked into deeply. Maybe your good intentions did not go well with your child. Here the challenge comes in- if you are in a mode of learning, to approach a situation in a better way. As it is a matter of your child, it's your responsibility to develop an appropriate thought-process in the child.

It is a popular thinking that almost all the problems of the world would be solved if human beings were more empathetic. It is POSSIBLE ONLY if parents develop **a skill** to communicate with their child.

According to the psychologists world over, there are four best parenting styles. These are the most important ones as these are commonly used in raising children.

The style in which the child is raised and communicates - plays a vital role in their development into maturity.

Yelling Mode

Majority of the parents have the most common way of addressing the children is yelling mode. The easiest of the methods is so abrupt, that even the parents realise it later.   This mode is the most famous and the easiest way of controlling the child. Parents believe that it is the easiest of the methods. My grown up children still can recall my yelling style. Though it is on the lighter side, it was never intentional. Whenever I was upset or in a hurry or even tired- this was my last resort. The aftermath was so horrible that it even made me cry, whenever I was alone. I felt guilty and cursed myself to be a failure as a parent.

Yelling mode is usually seen in common parenting. But we have to go into the main cause of it. The stress-level of the parents and the environment is the main cause of this mode. There is not even a single parent on this earth, who would intentionally yell at the child. So, here awareness of the types of parenting is important.

Types of Parenting

The four main parenting styles used in child psychology today are based on the work of *Diana Baumrind, a dev*elopmental psychologist and Stanford researchers Eleanor Maccoby and John Martin.

- Permissive

- Authoritative

- Neglectful

- Authoritarian

Authoritarian parenting

This type of parenting is commonly seen around us. Though this style is mostly preferred, as it brings out a desirable result in academics as well as in behavioural issues. The dire consequences of this kind is that the child is uncomfortable both socially and emotionally. Here the children are in continuous stress to satisfy their parents. The parents focus more on obedience, discipline and control rather than nurturing your child.

As this parenting is an extremely strict parenting style.Anxiety and self-doubt are the common issues which such children suffer with. These two factors create hindrance in establishing their personal identity. The reason that they have been conditioned in such a way, which has led them into a mindset which is pushing hard not to disappoint their parents.

Authoritarian parents place high demands on children and low levels of warmth. As a result,the children raised by these parents or guardians tend to struggle in all the spheres of their life. Be it emotionally, academically and socially.

Why do the AUTHORITARIAN Parenting need Coaches and Counsellors?

This is a hundred Dollar question. And the answer is that -

We need some external help, if we have to raise children with high self-esteem and better relationships. One cannot raise the next generation with the same mindset. Children are expected to always be obedient without much support.

They approach each and every aspect of the child in a similar manner. May it be- discipline or communication.

Characteristics of an authoritarian parenting style include-

1. <u>High Expectations</u>- They expect their children to have best results in academics, sports and other fields. They react so quickly and lack patience if their children do not come up to their expectations.

Why do the AUTHORITARIAN Parenting need Coaches and Counsellors?

This is a hundred Dollar question. And the answer is that -

We need some external help, if we have to raise children with high self-esteem and better relationships. One cannot raise the next generation with the same mindset. Children are expected to always be obedient without much support.

They approach each and every aspect of the child in a similar manner. May it be- discipline or communication.

Characteristics of an authoritarian parenting style include-

1. <u>High Expectations</u>- They expect their children to have best results in academics, sports and other fields. They react so quickly and lack patience if their children do not come up to their expectations.

2. <u>Punishments</u>- Misbehaviour or even petty childish issues are taken seriously by parents. In order to teach a lesson to their children they can even adopt severe ways of punishment. This is the main cause that such children are always unhappy and find it hard to express themselves with confidence.

3. <u>Lack of Communication</u>- This style of parenting has hardly any scope of open communication. These children are expected to follow guidelines without questioning. A void between parents and children is developed throughout life.

4. <u>Anger and anxiety</u>- The children brought up in an atmosphere of anger and anxiety, may struggle with low self-esteem. This itself prevents the child from growing up with a healthy mindset.

Outcome: Children tend to have negative development outcomes

1. Moderately -high levels of anxiety

2. Depressive symptoms

3. Withdrawal

4. Low self-esteem

5. Development of avoidant coping strategies

Authoritative parenting

The famous movie **The Lion King** (1994) is a fine example of authoritative parenting. In my opinion, each of us should see this movie once in a while. It has definitely given me some pointers, to check my parenting style and the mindset which we should develop to communicate with our children. The relationship between Simba and his Dad displays a sense of warmth, control and involvement of the parent in the child's life. This parenting style is more of a democratic kind- more of a mutual respect. In this way the parent makes sure that the child is provided with love and affection, thus trying to balance discipline along with.

Authoritative Parenting style is considered to be the most effective because it pays attention to the self-esteem of the child. The child brought up in a democratic environment grows up into a self-reliant and an optimistic individual. The most important is that he is in a positive mindset and as a result may have better outcomes.

Outcome - Children tend to have:

1. The best outcome in life as they are self-assured

2. A better self-esteem.

3. Excellent social skills

4. Overall better grades.

5. Independent outlook towards life.

6. The best outcome in life as they are self-assured

7. A better self-esteem.

8. Excellent social skills

9. Overall better grades

10. Independent outlook towards life.

Permissive Parenting

1. This type of parenting is easily understood by the name. The children have free reign.

2. The parent plays the role of a best friend instead of a parent.

3. Child grows up <u>without</u> a strong sense of self- discipline

4. Less academically motivated

5. Do not control or regulate their child's behaviour

6. Do not set limits or fail to be strict.

7. Responsive to their children's needs

8. Bribe their children with toys or gifts.

9. Dislike control and authority over their children

10.Permit them to become major decision-makers

Neglectful Parenting

The casual approach of humans will result in neglectful Parenting. It is referred to as uninvolved parenting which can be exemplified by an overall sense of indifference. Here they feel parenthood like a burden which results in limited engagement with their children and rules have no place in their lives. They avoid the children and stay uncaring, as they are struggling with their own issues.

<u>Summary of Chapter-7</u>

Communication

1. Treat your child with respect

2. Verbal and non verbal communication

3. Types of Parenting and their impact on the child's psychological and growth.

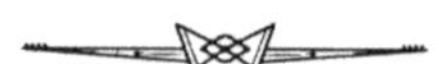

Chapter 8
Financial Literacy

"The school system will never teach you about money. It is designed to teach you to be an employee, which is important or a doctor or a lawyer or a specialist but never about money". - Robert Kiyosaki

When I was growing up, we were provided with a 'Bugni' or 'Gulak'.

In Hindi- it means a small pot shaped earthen container to collect money. In Western world these were made up of metallic material, but it had a special place in each child's life. It was not only a piggy bank but a place where our emotions settled. If a child wanted to give his parents, it was from his Piggy Bank. It worked as a magic to ingrain empathy in the children. And along with the children had to keep their spending urge in control.

" Financial Literacy is not an end in itself, but a step by step process. It begins in childhood and continues throughout a person's life all the way to retirement. Instilling the financial- literacy message in children is especially important, because they will carry it for the rest of their lives. The results of the survey are very encouraging, and we want to do our part to make sure all children develop and strengthen their financial -literacy skills".

Top Websites For Kids To Learn About Money

Kids and children can easily be taught financial literacy and its concept with the help of these websites:

1. Education 10x

2. Sense and Dollars

3. Money Sense

4. Juni Learning

5. Bankaroo

6. US Mint Coin Classroom

7. Hands on Banking

There can be a few steps vital for educating our children on Financial Planning.

1. **Money Management**- To manage small amounts of money,like pocket money. We as elders should allow the children to make minor decisions about thoughtful and right spending at an early age.

2 . **Activities**- Save, spend and earn can be taught to the child with the help of Games and with small amounts. They can learn budgeting by planning about their expenses like spending for toys, dresses, books etc. This kind of training in the kindergarten level definitely will help to keep their financial budget sorted.

3. **Value of Earning Money**- Children should be aware of the importance of the earned money. Their realisation that earning money is not so comfortable, will prevent them from wasting it. They can be given some money, such as doing some extra chores in the house. This would also make them understand the value of earning at the right time.

4. **Name of the currencies**- In their playtime or group activities the children can learn the names of various currencies which are being used in the different countries. The values of these will help them to understand more about the comparison of the expenditure in the different countries.

5. **Saving and investing**- These two things if learned and practised at an early age, are definitely going to reap long term results for the children. The correct method of saving and investing are the ladders of success towards financial security. This is a path leading towards financial planning.

6. Reckless spending - If the child is taught to plan his expenditure and earnings, this will prevent him from reckless spending habits. When the children understand this, the elders have an easy way with them. Many of the family tussles start with the money matters. All such issues will not occur as financial matters are sorted out in a habitual manner.

George Carl, Chairman of National CPA Financial Literacy Commission.

This depicts that we hardly invest in financial literacy in a meaningful way.

- The need of the hour is that our children should be trained to do the basic accounting, awareness about opening an account in the bank and why should the bills be paid on time.

The schools find it overwhelming to go for this kind of training, so the onus lies on the parents to take this aspect as early as possible.

- The parents can take their child along for visits to the bank, so that the kids get a slight familiarity with the space. It can be a methodical process, which can prove interesting for the parent and joyful for the child. The children are not born with a capacity to make sound financial decisions.

Let's walk through the process , so as to helping the parents from getting overwhelmed-

1. Train your child to make a budget for himself as early as possible. Whatever way he feels like.

2. Provide him a Piggy Bank, to curb over- spending.

3. to make financial decisions for himself, related to buying new toys or clothes etc. without you being critical.

4. Tell them stories about financial issues- in order to make them understand the importance of savings and investing.

5. Teach your child this COMMON Phrase-early in childhood.

'A penny saved is a penny earned'.

1. Instant gratification- This is the most important lesson which parents can train at their own level. One can begin with some delicious eatables or chocolates etc.

2. 'Early to bed, early to rise, makes a man healthy, wealthy and wise'.

- explain this phrase to your child by setting an example.

1. Formulate your own tricks and ideas to inculcate habits and behaviours in your child within your means.

2. Try to shed off your personal finance habits, which you have learned when you were a child.

3. Do not wait for your child to grow-up to take responsibility for his expenses.

Next, when the child enters middle school, the parents can take some steps further-

- BUDGETING- Teach your child how to learn **budgeting** by involving him, into daily household expenditure.

- Savings- Train him how to open a **Savings Account** and the various ways to operate it.

- Planning of Expenditure- Provide him with healthy tips to reduce the unnecessary **spendings**. In this way,he will learn the importance of Frugality. This will also need the indulgence of the parents to make the child understand the difference between miser and stingy.

- Let him understand the **basics of Bank loans**, so that it becomes easy for him to make decisions related to finances in the future.

- Concept of Compound Interest should be introduced to the child with the help of examples

- Introduce him to the share market, to how it works.

- An awareness about basic terminology related to finances can be introduced to the children with examples from their daily lives.

There are a few key things you should know about finance:

How to create a Budget?

How to track your expenses?

How to save money?

How to invest wisely?

By understanding these concepts, you'll be in a much better position to manage your finances and ensure the success of your business.

Summary of Chapter-8

Financial Literacy

1. Names of websites for awareness in parents.

2. Money management in early years of childhood.

3. Activities and Games

4. Value of earning money.

5. Names of the currencies

6. Train kids in saving and investing

7. To curb reckless spending

8. Visits to Banks and concepts related to it can help the child to manage their finances intelligently.

Chapter 9
Sex-Education

"Does sex education encourage sex?"

Many parents are afraid of talking about sex, in front of sex.

1. They start imagining that their children will be taking it as a permission for the teen to have sex .

2. To avoid embarrassing situations to discuss with their children, as it has been a Taboo for them in the Past.

3. The main idea of considering this topic of sex-education, in this first series of my book, is to make it clear for my readers about its importance.

4. It is healthy for the children to talk about sex with their parents and teachers.

5. If the people who take care of the all round development of their children, speak about sex with them.

6. The consequence of avoiding this topic would compel them to find out for themselves, and may even lead to distorted information from wrong sources.

7. Most people believe that talking about sexual information is a mixture of embarrassment and ignorance.

According to the **Dutch**, Education about Sexuality begins as early as age of four, when children receive lessons on relationships, appropriate touching and intimacy.

But what about the rest of the world, especially where we can find an increasing rate of sexual crimes. The research about sex-education has provided me with a clarity that until it remains a taboo in any society, it will keep taking the shape of crimes.

- Teach your child about Good Touch and Bad touch as early in childhood, as it is easy for him to raise his voice.

- To provide awareness to our kids about sex isn't easy, in any society.

- Unless we take this as our choice to provide our kids with it, we can save our children from sexual ignorance.

- Protecting oneself by getting molested and curbing the crime-rate of our society.

- Government cannot do much, if parents on their level do not take this responsibility of educating the children.

- All the efforts of the Government will go to waste, if the parents don't come forward for the sake of their own children.

Sex-education represents a different point of view of   children coming from different backgrounds and families. The Dutch approach to sex-education to be highly effective.

The Netherlands is the pioneer in sex-education for their next generation. The reason why this country has included sex-related education as early as to 4 years of age, is to protect their children from all sorts of crimes. It is proud of declaring that they are-

- One of the lowest rates of teen pregnancy in the world.

- Lowest rates of HIV

- Other STI' s- (Sexual Tranmitted Infections)

- Learn about safer sex.

- Lowest rate of sexual abuse in the world.

The world can learn a thoughtful lesson from the Dutch that-

- It is better to educate your children, before they find themselves in an awkward situation.

- This situation not only impacts the children physically but also can be hazardous for their mental and psychological growth.

- In many countries, it is a hush-hush situation and is a torturous state of mind where the child struggles individually.

Results of Sex-education -

1. Positive effects on personality of the child.

2. Reduce the rates of sexual activity

3. Reducing sexual risk-taking behaviours

4. Reduces STI/HIV Infection

5. Decreases ignorance.

6. It empowers children and young people to lead healthy, safe and productive lives.

7. To develop respectful social and sexual relationship

According to UNESCO, for Human beings to survive,
there are two basic needs-

1. Essential learning tools- such as literacy, oral expression, numeracy and problem-solving.

2. Basic Learning Content- such as knowledge, skills, values, and attitudes.

Researches have shown that the ignorance about sex-education, can even land the child in distraction and overwhelming situations. This may even impact his overall personality development. Lack of awareness may lead them into troubles, as no help is available to youth in conservative societies.

What made me ponder over this aspect of children, is thinking about the children vulnerable not only outside but in their Homes as well.

An episode on the Television hosted by Amir Khan shook me, where a young man revealed his own story. His mission was to create awareness in the audience. That day I understood how insecure the fearful boy might have felt. The worst part is when the child cannot even express their plight with their parents. As the parents do not believe them or snub them. Sometimes nears and dears can become villains for the child. It adds to the plight of the child, if the parents behave ignorant, when someone within your own family is trying to molest your child continuously. And you trust your relatives more than your child. I believe that it will be Hell-like in his own home.

TIPS FOR THE PARENTS

1. Beware of Strangers

No matter how old your child is -never leave your child alone with strangers nor with someone known.

2. Educate your child about sex.

Talk to him early in life about his sexual safety. Before   somebody else gives him distorted knowledge, it is better for you as a parent to provide him with the scientific awareness of this natural necessity in Humans.

3. Harmful consequences

Educate your child of the harmful impact of sexual activities- May lead to unwanted pregnancy, loss of faith in a pious institution of marriage and many other implications observed in the society during these modern times.

4. Self -Defence

Train him or her in Taekwondo or Karate etc. So that your child becomes self -confident and can fight against all odds.

5. Clear-cut instructions to your child

To be loud under such circumstances. Otherwise it may lead to further implications in life.

6. Develop trust in your CHILD

Let your child know that you are with him - no matter what. Develop faith in him that he should have a blind faith in your support. Do not make him feel guilty of any kind - only then he will confide in you.

Keep reminding him - "Come what may your Parents are there with you in all odds"

While I was going through my research , I came across a number of books by learned authors with a lot of professional experiences. But one of the books which resonated with my approach towards a blessed experience was

'Born to Thrive' - authored by Harvey Merrian. He has provided three simple steps which I think will be beneficial to those parents who are getting overwhelmed.

And I believe each one of us needs someone to help us in this journey. I think we are all in a Matrix. The one outside the matrix can see our situation in a different perspective. This is the reason why we look for Parenting Coaches. My clients come with a lot of stress of being Parents and a follow up brings them out of their awkward situation.

Step One – Politeness

As soon as the child enter the life of a family politeness ought to be consciously get in the members so the child inculcates the way of conversing and dealing with others. It is possible to raise children with zero harshness and zero punishment, and at the same time raise exceptionally smart, kind, and happy children.

According to Harvey, we can prevent anxiety, sibling rivalry, lack of motivation and confidence, bullying and many other insecurities of the child.

Step Two - Importance of Crying

"... the secretion of tears serves as a relief for suffering, and by as much as the weeping is more violent or hysterical, by so much will the relief be greater ...."

-

Charles Darwin, The Expression of the Emotions in Man and Animals, 1872

Crying functions as both a distress signal and an emotional healing process. Parents often mistake healing crying for a distress signal, and as a result they interrupt the healing. ***Born to Thrive!*** will show you how to support emotional healing and raise exceptionally resilient children, children who bounce right back from hurts and disappointments. If you are new to the approach, you will be amazed by the results.

Most importantly, crying can prevent psychological addictions and can help in good sleep. When the child sleeps after crying he goes into a deep sleep. This kind of sleep gives a soothing effect to his mental distress. Most of the time the parents are not able to find the reason of the crying of their child's crying.

Step Three – Less Control

Unnecessary control hampers children's development. It slows the development of judgement and wisdom, plus it triggers rebellion, turning what could have been a smooth, cooperative relationship into an adversarial one. ***Born to Thrive!*** Written by Harvey Marriem .will show you how to raise exceptionally cooperative, responsible, and self-motivated children. They will run their own lives so well that control would only get in their way.

<u>Summary of Chapter-9</u>

Sex-Education

1. Dutch education policy has set an example for the world, by providing sex-education at the early age of 4.

2. Tips for the parents to help their child to get educated at home itself.

3. It protects the child to receive a distorted information later, might lead them to harmful consequences.

Chapter 10
Workbook For Parents

WORKBOOK FOR PARENTS:

Q1. Mention 3 words to describe your Parenting Style ?

Q2. Your Biggest Strength as a Parent.

Q3. A situation in which you feel helpless as a parent.

Q4. One thing which you feel good about being a parent.

Q5. One thing which you feel guilty about as a parent,

Q6. Something about which you feel proud as a parent.

Q7. If your child comes home late after school. What will be your reaction?

Q8. What action would you take if your child quarrels with his classmate?

Q9. What would be your reaction if you child is scolded or punished by his teacher or someone elder?

Q10. If your child yells at you, what would be your response?

Chapter 11
Cyber Safety Needful for Children

What is Cyber?

As individuals, let's understand- Anything related to the internet or the use of modern ADVANCED systems and technologies.

In 2009,President Obama asked the Department of Homeland Security to create the **Stop.Think.Connect**. Campaign to help Americans understand the dangers that come with being online and the things we can do to protect ourselves and cyberthreats.

The most important issue of CYBERSECURITY for the Children has popped up these days. Parent in these modern times have to remember the following tips -

- Parents need to keep educating themselves in order to remain updated.

- Train and keep discussing with your child how to keep one's Personal information Private.

- Inform your child that while using the Internet should not share his name, address, Telephone number, birthday, Passwords and the name of his school.

- Keep reminding your child to never leave his mobile devices unattended and train him to keep a close eye on it.

- Create awareness to always keep his device locked by using a strong password.

- Important is to check that your child connects to the Internet, only when he needs to. His device should not be connected to Wi-Fi automatically.

- The apps should be checked by the parents before the child downloads any new app.

- The Computer teacher in the school should make sure that the child's awareness is updated. A clear understanding of cyberthreats in their networks should be taught.

- Let your child know the adverse consequences of talking to strangers online or never agree to meet anyone online or offline without your parents consent.

- Email offers for free like gifts, phones, earpods etc. should be informed first to your Parents. As these are tricks to lure you so that children give up their personal information to install malware or spyware.

Some common online issues kids face include:

-Cyber predators

Cyber predators are people who search online for other people in order to use, control or harm them in some way.

-Cyber Bullying

Cyberbullying is the electronic posting of disturbing messages about the child so that the child gets disturbed and reveals more about himself and gets trapped.

-Identity Theft

It is the illegal use of personal information in order to steal money or credit.

Reason for awareness in the children about cybersecurity is that during Covid days they were on INTERNET for their school and tution classes. Thus providing an easy access for them.

At that time not only the children but also the grown ups were using the internet .

The Campaign - 'Stop.Think.Connect.' has provided some effective TIPS for the Kids.

1. Campaign of this kind is an eye-opener for the parents, in which they are helped to remain fully aware.

2. According to their researches-

- Kids ages 8-18 spend 7 hours and 38 minutes per day online

- If the child sleeps 8 hours per night that means one half of the time that he or she is awake is spent online-

33% online

33%offline

33% sleep

3. These kinds of Campaigns are the need of the hour so that our generation does not fall into trouble.

DOXING

As I was going through an article by Colette Bernard. In this she has explained about Doxing or Doxxing. According to her research this is a scary problem that can put your family members and their real identity in danger. Being Doxed is a form of cyberbullying. She has given her piece of advice that as parents we should talk to them about it.

Teach your child what Doxing is and how it can harm them.

- **Strong Password**

Make sure they use a strong password and have a different one for every gaming account.

- **Fake name and the email address**

Help your child and train him to use a fake name and email address on social media.

- **Location Service to be turned off**

Help your child to turn off the location services in the setting of the device. In this way a doxxer can be prevented.

<u>Summary of Chapter 11</u>

Cyber Safety

1. On the whole we cannot force the child to stay away from internet but we as parents, need to educate them well.

2. Awareness about its pros and cons is the need of the hour.

3. Inculcating a sense of responsibility in the child is needed.

Chapter 12

Self-Care: Most Needed for all the Parent

In the beginning of the book, my purpose was to provide an awareness for the parents who want some preparation for their Parenthood. As we go through prior training to enter our work place, we are excited to learn during our internship. Why not take Parenting as a challenge with complete head and heart into it. The second challenge is rather more complex, because we have to nurture a human soul. There are no replays in this journey. Now the question in the mind of the reader is then maybe parenting is overwhelming? Yes it is , but it is also a mixed bag of joy mixed with splashes of uncertainty and surprises. This amalgamation is what PARENTING is all about. This experience is felt by only those blessed individuals who are lucky enough to get the privilege of Parenthood.

The beauty of parenting is that- it is different for each individual. And again I would stress that there are several factors which influence the style of Parenting. Generation to generation the traits are carried along . On this journey, they get disrupted while some get modified or rectified.

You may be wondering that when all was well-stated earlier, then why this Topic on Self-care now.

So, it is obvious that work well started is half done, but do you think everything goes according to our wishes or desires? Maybe some things but not all. Like our families and the people around may not cooperate or some health issues may hinder our efforts. There is a list of unavoidable circumstances in our lives. Sometimes even our own nature, habits and attitudes also disrupt our Parenting journey to some extent.

The worst part is that our approach towards our children boomerangs on us. This puts us in an unavoidable situation that we become enemies of our children. This is the last thing we would ever wish for in our lives.

There are thousands of factors which affect the Parent-child relation-ship. Right from the prenatal stage to adulthood of the child, there are several processes which influence the child during his growth. Even if how careful and aware the parent is, there are some or the other aspects of the personality of the child which remains recessive all through his childhood. A parent cannot control or check each one of these. And it is Ok with it, here the parent cannot be blamed as the child has not only been trained and nurtured by you. The family members, the society, the genes and the child's own nature play separate roles in his life.

1. The parents have to look after themselves well to take care of their child in a healthy manner.

2. A child learns life-skills by observing his/her parents.

3. Self-care is maintaining balance between mind and body.

4. Meditation, exercise and a healthy diet are the ones which need priority, rest will follow.

5. Parenting is a job similar to a CEO of a company. If we treat it in this manner we would never go wrong.

6. Element of Joy and Long-Term Relationship needs to be nurtured at each step.

7. Parenting Journey can be approached in a manner similar to tracking or mountaineering- which is not easy but along with excitement and fond memories which remain with us to be cherished later.

1. Campaign of this kind is an eye-opener for the parents, in which they are helped to remain fully aware.

2. According to their researches-

- Kids ages 8-18 spend 7 hOURS and 38 minutes per day online

- If the child sleeps 8 hours per night that means one half of the time that he or she is awake is spent online-

33% online

33%offline

33% sleep

3. These kinds of Campaigns are the need of the hour so that our generation does not fall into trouble.

Summary of Chapter-12

1. Self-care for parents is the most important.

2. Parents to act as CEO's at home providing a democratic as well as loving environment.

3. Spread happiness in the child's life with balance is important.

4. Leaving this Earth with responsible citizens

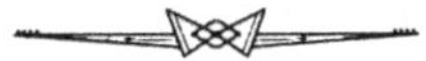

Copyright

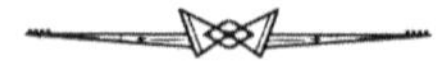